Contents

Foreword

I encouraged Michael to write this book because I have always found him to be an inspiring figure. Even with his epilepsy, he has always been someone who can make me forget about his condition. When we first started dating, he was worried that his epilepsy would be a burden for me and that I would want to end our relationship. However, I told him that I was not afraid of epilepsy and that I had experience with it from someone I went to school with.

While it can be scary to witness someone having a seizure, it is important to know how to react and ensure the safety of both the person with epilepsy and those around them. Too often, people overreact and call for an ambulance right away, when in reality the best thing to do is just let the person rest because it wears their body out. It is only necessary to call an ambulance if someone is having multiple seizures. With Michael's book, I hope that more people will become informed about epilepsy and learn how to properly handle seizures.

Our cat displayed remarkable intuition when it came to Michael's seizures. She would circle around him, detecting the signs before anyone else. Once Michael had the seizure, she would quietly go and lay down on the bed beside him, a comforting presence in the room. She would then remain by his side, a loyal companion, until he got back up. It was really sweet. Animals sense that. It was touching to witness how in tune our pets can be with our emotions and physical well-being.

Michael's epilepsy has never deterred him from pursuing his goals and aspirations. Despite being faced with this challenge, he has gone above and beyond his duties as an employee by acquiring three additional pharmacy licenses in just one year at the request of his employer. When most people are very young, they are allowed five trials, and most of them take up to five. Being in his sixties, he passed everyone of them immediately. He doesn't see how smart he is; he has so much to offer and inspire people.

I recently had a customer that I was just starting to do business with. I had called him to give him some information, and I heard a woman speaking in the background, "Just a minute, Carol, just a minute". After a little bit, he got back. I asked if he was okay, and he said he just had a seizure, and it was his nurse who had spoken earlier.

I told him my husband is an epileptic and he is a pharmacist, so he proceeded to tell me more details about his situation, and I gave him a little snippet of Mike's story. I called him a couple of times and wasn't hearing back from him, and I was very concerned. So, I sent him an email and put the subject line "inspiration" and he read the little snippet and told me he had just had another seizure the night before and was in the hospital flipping through his phone when he came across my email and saw the subject line saying "inspiration". He said, "Carol, you sent that to me, and I read that in one of my darkest moments".

I introduced him to Michael, and he was able to share some of his past information with him to let him know he was not alone in the world. It really helped this gentleman out a lot, and I know there are other people that Michael can inspire.

Michael and I are 21 years old in marriage, and he has not had a grand mal seizure in 15 years. He told me that I'd contributed to that, and I told him he could not have ever given me a finer compliment than that.

I have always been one to take care of those around me, and Michael is no exception. I make it a point to ensure that he is well taken care of and that all of his needs are met. One aspect of his health that I worry about in particular is his nutrition. I know that when he was single, he had a tendency to skip meals or eat poorly, which resulted in him losing weight and becoming quite thin.

To combat this, I take great care in planning out our meals every day. I ensure that he is getting all the essential nutrients he needs to stay healthy and strong. I make sure that our meals are well-balanced and contain plenty of vegetables, proteins, and healthy fats. I also try to limit our intake of processed and unhealthy foods as much as possible.

Aside from his nutrition, another important aspect of his health that I focus on is his rest. I know that he has a tendency to work long hours and push himself too hard. When he is tired, I encourage him to rest and take breaks throughout the day. I also make sure that he is getting enough sleep at night and that he is comfortable and relaxed in bed.

All of my efforts seem to be paying off, as he has not had any seizures recently. He has expressed how grateful he is for everything that I do and how much my actions have contributed to his overall wellbeing. Knowing that I am making a positive impact on his health gives me a great sense of fulfillment, and I feel happy to be able to contribute to his health and happiness in such a meaningful way.

Once, he came home and shared with me how a mother with a child who had been diagnosed with epilepsy came to the pharmacy and how she seemed to be filled with despair and hopelessness, acting like it's a death sentence. He took the opportunity to speak with the child privately and disclosed that he himself had been epileptic since he was 9 years old and was now a pharmacist. By sharing his journey, he aimed to give hope and help the child realize that there was light at the end of the tunnel—a giant, bright light to embrace. His compassionate words and actions could inspire more people, especially young children who were dealing with a similar diagnosis.

He literally makes me forget that he is an epileptic, and when I tell people that my husband's an epileptic, they're like "Oh, I'm sorry". Then I go, "There's nothing to be sorry about." He's an achiever, and he has never stopped achieving. I just want him to share his story because he is such a positive inspiration. I think he can do good for a lot of people, and that's why I wanted him to write this story.

Carol McQueen

Introduction

This book holds a singular purpose for me: to inspire anyone who's been told, time and time again, that there are things out of their grasp, or perhaps they've started believing it themselves. It is here to inspire and motivate, urging you to push against the limits that might have been set by others or even by your own doubts. It's like a beacon, casting light on the boundless possibilities within each reader and igniting a sense of empowerment and hope.

So, my dear reader, I urge you to take hold of this book with both hands and allow its wisdom to seep into your soul. Let the words within these pages ignite a fire within you, a fire that burns with passion, inspiration, and a strong sense of self-belief. And as you read on, remember that you are not alone in your struggles. We all face challenges in life, but it is how we rise above them that define us.

So, let this book be your guide, your counselor, and your friend. Let it help you break through the limitations that others or even your own doubts have placed on you. Let it be a source of inspiration and hope as you navigate the ups and downs of life.

Remember, the path to success is not always smooth, but with perseverance, determination, and a strong sense of self-belief, you can achieve anything you set your mind to. So, embrace your inner strength, tap into your limitless potential, and go forth to create the life you have always dreamed of. This book is here to remind you that anything is possible if you believe in yourself. Let it be the catalyst that sparks a transformation in your life, and may it inspire you to soar to new heights of greatness.

As you begin this journey through the pages of my story, I invite you to walk alongside me and experience the challenges that I have faced head-on with unwavering resilience and unyielding resolve. Living with epilepsy has been an ever-present battle, but one that I have refused to let define my life. Instead, I have chosen to confront it head-on, and my story is a testament to the fact that it is possible to live a rich, fulfilling, and regular life even in the face of adversity.

At times, epilepsy can seem like a daunting presence, a force that threatens to upend your sense of well-being and stability. The seizures can be sudden and unpredictable, leaving you feeling vulnerable and helpless. However, I have learned that the key to overcoming this condition is to recognize that it is not the end of the road. It does not have to define who you are or hold you back from achieving your goals and dreams.

Through my story, I hope to inspire others to take control of their lives and refuse to allow epilepsy, or any other condition, to limit their potential. I have lived a life filled with twists, turns, and unexpected challenges, but I have never lost sight of my goals or my determination to succeed. With the strength and support of my loved ones, I have been able to face each obstacle with courage and conviction.

As you journey with me, you will witness the highs and lows of living with epilepsy. You will see how I have learned to manage my symptoms and live a fulfilling life, despite the challenges I have faced. You will see that it is possible to build a life filled with joy, purpose, and meaning, even in the face of adversity.

So come with me on this journey. Witness my triumphs and setbacks, and discover for yourself that epilepsy is not the end of the road. With resilience, determination, and a never-give-up attitude, anything is possible, and a rich, fulfilling, and regular life is within your reach.

Chapter 1

Lufkin Memorial Hospital was located in a quiet part of Lufkin, Texas, USA. It was a small, community-based facility that served the people of Lufkin, Texas, and the surrounding areas. The environment was quiet and peaceful, very different from the bustling city we see today. The hospital was a safe haven, a place where life moved at a slower pace and where kindness and care were at the heart of everything.

On a sunny Thursday, the 30th of October in 1958, I, Michael McQueen, was born at the hospital during lunchtime. After taking my first breath, my grandmother cradled me in her warm and loving arms before taking me to her home. My maternal grandparents, Grandma Mae and Grandpa O.D., who were 48 and 52, respectively, warmly welcomed me into their world.

My parents had tied the knot in February of 1958, and I was born in October of that same year. This means that I was conceived just a few months after their marriage. Although some individuals may view this as evidence that I was not planned, I have never felt like an accident. Rather, I have always felt loved and valued by my parents.

My dad, Jimmy McQueen, was a dedicated truck driver. He often arrived home in his massive 18-wheeler truck. He spent long hours driving those enormous machines, occasionally even making trips all the way up to Canada. I distinctly remember glimpsing in the glove compartment of his truck, and I would imagine finding candy in there too. Every Friday evening, we would make our way to the racetrack.

During the late 1950s, the trucking industry in the United States was experiencing a period of significant growth. With the construction of the interstate highway system underway, trucking companies were expanding their routes and increasing their fleets. The demand for truck drivers, like Jimmy McQueen, was high, and many people like him found steady employment and job security in this field.

As a truck driver in the 1950s, my dad usually had to navigate older, narrow roads and bridges that were not always designed for a large vehicle like an 18-wheeler. This required a high level of skill and concentration, especially when traveling long distances. Additionally, as a driver making trips to Canada, he would often have had to deal with border crossings and international regulations.

Overall, my dad's job as a truck driver was physically demanding and required a great deal of dedication and hard work. Despite the challenges, he was committed to his profession, and his work helped contribute to the growth of the trucking industry during a significant period in American history in its own little way.

It was therefore heartbreaking to hear that just merely three years after my birth, my father passed away. My dad was an amazing person, and he had a close relationship with his aunts from the McQueen family. They were doting and loving towards him, always showering him with affection and attention. It was no secret that he was their favorite nephew, and they would often spoil him with gifts and treats.

When my dad passed away, I couldn't help but feel a deep sense of loss. He was such an important figure in my life, and the thought of not having him around anymore was heartbreaking. It is interesting that I later took his place as my favorite nephew.

Although his aunts had all passed away, I knew that they had lived long and full lives. In fact, I believe that two of them have reached the impressive milestone of 100 years old. The third aunt had surpassed that, living to be an incredible 104 years of age. It was a testament to the strength and resilience of the McQueen family, and their longevity was something to admire.

At the age of five, my mom, Nancy, had to leave Lufkin for Houston in search of work, leaving me with my grandparents. In the early 1960s, the economy of Lufkin, a small town in Texas, was struggling. Opportunities for employment were scarce, and many families were struggling to make ends meet. This led to a wave of migration from Lufkin to larger cities like Houston, where job opportunities were more abundant.

For families like mine, this meant making a difficult decision. My mother, Nancy, had to leave me with my grandparents in Lufkin in order to search for work in Houston. This was not an uncommon situation, as parents often had to make sacrifices in order to provide for their families during this time.

The decade of the 1960s was a time of great change in the United States. The civil rights movement was gaining momentum, and the country was still reeling from the assassination of President John F. Kennedy. It was also a time of great economic growth, but this growth was not evenly distributed across the country.

By leaving Lufkin for Houston, my mother was part of a larger trend of migration that was shaping the economic and social landscape of the United States. This decision would have a profound impact on my life, as I would come to live with my grandparents and grow up in a different environment from the one I believe my mother had initially intended for me.

It was in Houston that she eventually decided to get married again, and her wedding was held in Lufkin. To my surprise, I was chosen to be their ring bearer, and this was a significant moment for my stepdad, who showed his acceptance of me and my mom. As time went on, my mom and stepdad welcomed two little girls into the world, and they became my half-sisters.

Our family has a unique dynamic, and it's something I cherish. You see, every one of us, including my siblings, were born in October, and there's a six-year gap between each of our birthdays. This makes our family a blend of various ages and backgrounds, but it also creates a special bond among us, especially during our birthday month.

After the wedding, however, I did not move in with my new family. I chose to stay with my wonderful grandparents. After my dad passed away and my mom left for Houston, it was my dear grandparents who stepped in as my legal guardians. I typically stayed in touch with my mother through phone conversations, and every now and then, she would come to visit us.

I was fortunate enough to grow up surrounded by children who were all around the same age as me. This meant that there was hardly ever a dull moment, as we always had someone to play with and something to do. One of our favorite things to do was play sports, especially football and basketball. We would often spend hours outside, running around and working up a sweat as we tried to outdo each other on the field or court.

It was a time when children played outside without the distractions of smartphones and other modern technology. Our neighborhood was considered safe, and our parents didn't have to worry too much about us playing outside for hours on end. Sports were a big part of our lives, with football and basketball being the most popular among our group. It was a carefree time in our lives, and I enjoyed every minute of it.

Even on rainy days, we would find a way to have fun together. We would retreat to someone's house and pull out board games or chess boards, challenging each other to intense matches that could last for hours on end. These games were a great way to bond and spend time together, even when the weather was less than ideal.

Riding my bike around the neighborhood was one of my favorite things to do as a child. I was never afraid of going too far or getting lost, as I loved the sense of freedom and independence that came with navigating the streets on my own. I even used to teach tennis lessons, passing on my love of sports and physical activity to others who were eager to learn.

During that period of my life, one of the individuals who became incredibly close to me was someone who stood out as a unique character to many. Possessing a remarkable intellect, he effortlessly aced all his subjects, yet he grappled with a fundamental skill: riding a bicycle. It struck me as a curious contrast. Determined to help him overcome this challenge, I took it upon myself to teach him how to ride a bicycle. We dedicated countless hours, with me patiently providing guidance as he navigated the uneven terrain, wobbling and stumbling along the way.

Finally, after a series of small victories and a heap of perseverance, he achieved the feat of biking with the finesse of a seasoned pro like the other kids in the environment. Seeing the radiant smile that spread across his face and sensing the palpable surge of accomplishment that emanated from him was an experience that left an indelible mark on me. It served as a powerful reminder that every individual harbors their unique set of strengths and vulnerabilities, regardless of how capable or intelligent they may appear to the world. This shared journey underscored the beauty of embracing diversity in abilities and the profound impact that support and encouragement can have on one's path to triumph.

Before I was born, my grandparents used to run a grocery store. They were still running the store when my dad, who worked at Hick's gas station across the street, met my mom. I remember spending time at the grocery store before my dad passed away. It was located beside a place called Top Burger, where I would buy a giant burger for 25 cents.

My grandparents later sold the store and got into the car business. As I grew up, my grandfather always owned a purple Willis Jeep with yellow wheels. I learned how to drive in that Jeep when I was only ten years old by driving it around the car lot.

So, my grandfather owned a used car lot, where he'd spend his days wheeling and dealing with all sorts of vehicles. It was like a playground for him, filled with engines roaring and potential customers milling about. And my grandmother sold world-book encyclopedias. So, by no means, were we wealthy.

Despite their humble means, they worked tirelessly to provide for me, ensuring that I had all that I needed to grow up. While their income may have been considered average at best, the wealth of their affection and guidance made my childhood nothing short of extraordinary. They instilled in me values that went far beyond material wealth.

Mamaw and Papaw—those were the names I called them. They were so much more than just grandparents; they were my guides and biggest supporters. Reflecting on it now, I realize what an immense blessing it was to have them by my side. They imparted invaluable life lessons, emphasizing the significance of doing what's right, even in the face of challenges.

I was generally a well-behaved child. I mostly listened to my grandparents and followed their instructions. The only time I can remember getting in trouble was when we were on vacation, and my grandpa gave me a good whipping. He made sure I understood the lesson he was trying to teach.

Papaw, my maternal grandfather, also taught me the power of facing life head-on, shoulders squared. These teachings became the cornerstone of my character as I grew older. Their love and counsel shaped me into the person I am today. They were, without a doubt, truly exceptional.

Every single Sunday, without fail, my grandparents and I made our way to church. I absolutely loved it. Our church, while small with only about 34 members, felt like a close-knit family. Those Sundays were like treasures, moments I held dear.

I remember the only birthday party I ever had. It was unlike any other party that I had ever been to or would ever attend again. I was still little then, and my Sunday school teacher from church, Nancy, dressed up as a witch. It was the highlight of the party for me, and I could feel her love and care for me in every detail of the party. She put so much thought and effort into creating a fun and magical experience for everyone.

Our church, Keltys Methodist Church, had been a staple in our small community for as long as anyone could remember. It was a place where families came to worship, children learned about God, and everyone was welcomed with open arms.

As time went on, the landscape of the church began to change. Other churches in the area started merging, and soon enough, our church became Keltys United Methodist Church. While the changes may seem small, they held a lot of significance for those of us who had grown up attending church.

During my time at Keltys United Methodist Church, I was baptized. At the time, I didn't believe in being sprinkled to be baptized. I wanted the full experience of being submerged, just as Jesus had been in the river Jordan. So, I asked the preacher to take me to a Baptist church to undergo the baptismal ceremony.

The experience was definitely memorable, but not exactly in the way I had hoped. The preacher at the Baptist Church was new to the idea of submerging people for baptism, and I was his first. Suffice it to say, I almost ended up drowning! Looking back on it now, it's a funny memory and one that I cherish as a reminder of the importance of community and faith in our lives.

Experiencing a community where people genuinely cared for each other was a remarkable occurrence. Through attending a small church, I realized the tremendous influence of togetherness and the strength that emerges from a shared faith. These moments, characterized by common convictions and emotional connections, were the most enjoyable parts of my week.

Chapter 2

As I look back on my early years, the memories of Kurth Elementary School flood my mind. There were these instances when I'd find myself in a sort of trance for about five seconds. It was as if I took a quick mental vacation. I'm sure my teachers probably thought I was daydreaming during those moments. It happened quite often, so much so that my grandmother thought it was time to see a local doctor.

But looking back on it now, I can see that these episodes were more than just normal moments of confusion or disorientation. They were seizures, plain and simple. And they were happening more frequently than I even realized. At times, they occurred every single day, yet those episodes were so brief that they were easy to brush aside as nothing more than momentary lapses in concentration.

I was around 4th or 5th grade back then, and to be honest, I didn't quite grasp the full picture of what was going on. All I sensed was that there was something a bit different about what I was experiencing.

The local doctor my grandma took me to see, after checking me over, said we needed to head to the Houston Medical Center. When we arrived, I was subjected to a barrage of tests and examinations. It was overwhelming, to say the least. Finally, the doctor called my grandmother and me into his office to discuss his findings. And that's when he told me the news—I had epilepsy.

The doctor explained that epilepsy is a neurological disorder that causes seizures. He also told me that it is a chronic condition that cannot be cured but can be managed with medication. He prescribed me medication to help control my seizures and explained how to take it and when to take it.

My grandmother was shocked and saddened by the news, and I could see the worry on her face. The doctor reassured her that with proper treatment and management, epilepsy can be controlled, and people with epilepsy can live full and productive lives.

The doctor also explained that I would need to make some lifestyle adjustments, such as getting enough sleep, avoiding triggers that cause seizures, and not engaging in certain activities that could be dangerous if I were to have a seizure.

Leaving the doctor's office, my head was spinning with all of the new information I had just received. I felt overwhelmed and scared. It was difficult for me to process that I had a chronic medical condition that would require ongoing management and care.

I was only 10 years old, and I had no idea what that meant, but the way the doctor spoke about it made me feel like it was something terrible. For a moment, I felt myself giving in to the fear that was gnawing at me. But then I saw my grandmother's unwavering support, and I knew I couldn't let this diagnosis defeat me. My spirit, though shaken, was unbroken. I was determined to face this challenge head-on and prove to everyone, including myself, that epilepsy wouldn't define me.

From that moment on, my journey took a sudden turn. There were medications to manage, doctor's appointments to attend, and lifestyle changes to make. But through it all, I held on to my determination and resilience. I refused to let epilepsy be the end of me; instead, I saw it as an opportunity to grow and learn.

Adjusting to life with epilepsy was not easy, but with the support of my family and healthcare professionals, I was able to control my seizures and live a full and active life. It took time, but eventually, I learned that having epilepsy did not define me. With the encouraging words of the doctor and my grandparents in mind, I continued on my life journey.

It wasn't always a breeze. There were times when the road got rough, but I pressed on. I was resolute in my mission to show not only myself but also the world that I could overcome any challenge, even epilepsy. This determination became my driving force, propelling me forward through every obstacle that stood in my path. Along the way, I learned that resilience and unwavering belief in oneself can be powerful tools in the face of adversity.

As a young child, I loved to spend my days playing outside with my friends in our yard. However, every now and then, my grandma would suddenly appear at the door and interrupt our game. With a worried look on her face, she would tell me to come inside, saying that I was going to have a seizure.

For me, these words were like a death sentence. I would feel a mixture of fear and shame, knowing that my friends would hear my grandma's warning and see me being taken away from our game. In my mind, having a seizure was a sign of weakness and vulnerability, something that I didn't want my friends to witness or think less of me for.

At that moment, I would have preferred to have the seizure than to face the embarrassment of being seen as different or abnormal. It wasn't until much later in life that I learned to accept my epilepsy and embrace the support of my loved ones, including my grandma. But in those early days, all I could think about was how much I wanted to be like everyone else, even if it meant putting my own health at risk.

As I got older, my encounters with epilepsy grew more complex. It had begun when I was just 10 with petit mal seizures, a surreal pause in the midst of reality. But time rolled on, and so did my condition. The seizures transformed into grand mal seizures, which were different and much more intense. These episodes were a whirlwind of intensity, shaking me to my core. Each one was a stark reminder of the unpredictability that epilepsy brought into my life. But I held on, knowing that, with the support of my family, I could face whatever came my way.

During a grand mal seizure, everything goes dark. It's like all the lights in my mind shut off. My muscles, once at ease, now seem to contract and then relax again. It's a strange sensation, this internal struggle, and it leaves me feeling powerless and disconnected from my own body. The world outside blurs into a chaotic whirlwind of incomprehensible sights and sounds. Time loses its regular beat; seconds stretch and twist, making each moment feel like an eternity.

It's a disconcerting feeling to be trapped in this surreal realm where nothing seems quite real or tangible.

As the storm rages on, there's a peculiar mix of fear and resignation. I hold on, knowing that there's nothing I can do but wait for it to pass. It's a terrifying experience, feeling so utterly out of control, yet I've learned to trust that eventually the lights will flicker back to life and I'll find myself back in the world I know.

Emerging from a grand mal seizure is like waking from a turbulent dream. When I finally come back to myself, there's always a lingering sense of confusion; everything is both familiar and strange. There are times when I'd discover myself a little worse for wear, with no recollection of how it came to be; I'd find myself a bit banged up or bruised.

These incidents brought to light the unpredictable challenges that come with epilepsy. One particularly memorable occasion involved a seizure that left my shoulder broken and dislocated. Strangely, the pain only hit me as I started to regain consciousness. My body felt out of sync, struggling to catch up with the sudden shift.

Having experienced multiple injuries and medical emergencies, including receiving a staggering 21 stitches across my eye, breaking and dislocating my shoulder, I must admit that my body has been through quite a lot.

At times, my seizures would get the better of me, and I remember those instances when I would unintentionally punch holes in the sheetrock. It wasn't a way to release pent-up frustration, as some might assume. Rather, it was a physical manifestation of my seizures. I always made sure to let people know to give me some space if they ever saw me in the midst of a seizure. It wasn't because I wanted to cause harm, but rather, in that state, I understood I might unintentionally lash out. This experience taught me the vital importance of empathy and the value of a strong support system.

As someone with a history of seizures, I knew that I had to approach sports and physical activities with caution in order to avoid putting myself in danger. Though I was passionate about sports, I knew that each engagement carried a certain level of excitement and exertion that could potentially trigger a seizure. Therefore, it was always a delicate balance to strike between pursuing my athletic interests and taking the necessary precautions to keep myself safe.

Those early years of my life were marked by the constant presence of seizures. They were unpredictable and would strike without any warning, leaving me bewildered and disoriented. I remember the panic that would set in as I felt the seizure coming on and the fear that would consume me as I was rushed to the hospital. As we drove closer and closer to the emergency room, the cloud of confusion would slowly lift, and I was left piecing together my surroundings.

In those moments, I was acutely aware of my vulnerability. I was just a young person, grappling with something that seemed far beyond my control. The experience of a seizure was both physically and emotionally jarring. I would emerge feeling shaky and disoriented, struggling to remember where I was or what had just happened. It was a lonely and unnerving experience, and one that left me feeling uncertain about the future.

Once the doctors had assessed my condition, I was allowed to return home. But even then, I usually found it hard to shake the anxiety that had taken hold of me.

Living with epilepsy was never easy for me. As I grew up, I faced several challenges that tested my strength and resilience. Despite my best efforts, I couldn't always control the way my body reacted during a seizure. It was a constant source of frustration and embarrassment for me.

One of the toughest things to deal with was the fact that my bladder would let go when I had a seizure. It was something that happened regularly, and it was incredibly humiliating. As a child, I remember feeling embarrassed when it happened at school and feeling like I was different from the other kids because of it.

As I grew older, the embarrassment didn't fade away because I continued to experience it. One time, I went to a friend's house to play board games like chess, and I had a seizure while sitting there. I soiled their furniture in the process, and that was hard for me mentally, but my friend and his parents never said anything. I knew they were aware of my situation at the time.

It wasn't just the physical aspect of it that was difficult to deal with; it was also my fear of how others perceived me. I knew people might notice, but they didn't say anything. It made me wonder if they were silently judging me. Maybe they thought I was gross, weak, or incapable. Maybe they pitied me.

It was a real inner battle because I couldn't help but wonder what people were really thinking about me. I wanted to be seen as normal and capable, but the reality was that my condition made that difficult. But as time went on, I realized that my fears were mostly unwarranted. Most people were more understanding than I gave them credit for. They saw past the seizures and accepted me for who I was. It was a lesson in acceptance and self-love. I couldn't control my seizures, but I could control how I viewed myself and my condition.

As time went on, I found a way to handle these episodes with more grace and confidence. I came to understand that they were a part of me, but they didn't define who I was. With the unwavering support of my family, I mustered the strength to confront each seizure with courage. They taught me that it's perfectly normal to feel scared, yet it's crucial to keep pressing forward.

Chapter 3

As I look back on those early years after learning about my epilepsy, it's clear that my grandma and grandpa were my true champions. They devoted endless hours to taking me to various doctors, chiropractors, and even preachers, all in pursuit of a way to help me. Their determination and unwavering support were nothing short of extraordinary. They never saw me as a burden, even though dealing with my condition was undoubtedly a challenge. Their love for me knew no bounds, and I am forever grateful for their selflessness. Their actions spoke volumes, showing me that I was cherished beyond measure. I now understand how incredibly fortunate I was to have had them by my side.

I can still recall those lengthy drives to various places, all in pursuit of something that could make a positive change. My grandma never showed impatience or fatigue. Her commitment to my well-being was steadfast. It felt like she would travel to the farthest corners of the earth if it meant a chance for me to lead a better, more comfortable life. Her unwavering support became the cornerstone of my journey towards healing and acceptance.

We also explored healing through two religious lines. During the late 1960s, epilepsy was still widely misunderstood and stigmatized. Medical knowledge regarding the disorder was limited, and many doctors were simply not equipped to properly diagnose and treat epilepsy. This meant that many people like myself, who were suffering from seizures, were often misdiagnosed or labeled as mentally impaired.

I sought out the best epileptic doctor in the world to try and get to the bottom of my condition. Unfortunately, even this highly esteemed professional was unable to find anything physically wrong with me. Frustrated and unsure of what else to do, she made the decision to diagnose me as being retarded.

To compound matters, she prescribed a medication called Tridion, which was considered a high-dose drug at the time. This drug was used to treat a range of conditions, including epilepsy, but it was later found to be toxic to the retina. Because of this, Tridion is no longer available on the market today.

This medication, which I began taking, contained elements that adversely affected my eyes, further complicating matters. I believed it would be the solution to my struggles; however, it brought about its own set of challenges. I still attended school and even engaged in sports, despite my limited vision. I could only discern the outline of the football as I caught it, but I did not let my condition hinder me.

The fact that a doctor could make such an incorrect and damaging diagnosis back then underscores just how limited medical knowledge was about neurological disorders like epilepsy at the time. The stigma surrounding epilepsy also meant that many people like me were unfairly labeled as being mentally deficient simply because of our condition.

Consequently, my doctors decided to discontinue that medication. They recommended chiropractic treatment, which meant regular visits to a specialist three times a week. I was willing to explore any possibility that might offer me some relief, so I went for it with my grandparents by my side. And my grandma drove me 40 miles one way, three times a week, in hopes that a chiropractor could provide a remedy.

Around the age of 15 or 16, something really frightening happened to me. It is called status epilepticus, which is just a fancy term for when seizures keep coming, one after the other. It was like being trapped in a never-ending cycle. I found myself in the hospital, where they administered medication to curb the seizures, and this went on for a couple of days.

While all this was going on, I could hear what the doctor was saying, but when I tried to respond, my words got all jumbled up. It was incredibly frustrating because, even though I knew what I wanted to say, it came out in a way that made no sense to anyone. It was almost like speaking a different language, or as if I was speaking in tongues.

Being in that situation was not easy, but it also showed me just how strong and determined I could be. Even when things got incredibly hard, I didn't give up. I kept pushing forward, and eventually, things started to improve. It was a huge lesson for me about the power of determination and not letting challenges define who I am.

After that experience, I learned to treasure moments of calm and stability even more. It made me realize that even when things seem incredibly tough, there's always a way to push through and come out stronger on the other side; there's always a way to find balance and keep moving forward. It's a lesson that's stuck with me all my life, a reminder that I can overcome anything as long as I believe in myself and keep moving forward.

A shift in medication followed this particularly severe episode called "status epilepticus". It became evident that the chiropractic sessions alone couldn't do the trick. That's when I sought help from Dr. Rivera at the medical center in Houston. He recommended a different kind of medication, and fortunately, it seemed to have a positive impact. It was a challenging journey, marked by trials and experiments to discover what suited me best. However, amidst it all, I clung to the hope that one day I'd stumble upon the perfect combination of treatments to leave those seizures in the rearview.

At the hospital, I went through a bunch of tests. The doctors poked and prodded, trying to figure out what was going on inside my brain. But after all those tests, they still didn't have any answers. No weird spots, no strange marks—nothing. One doctor thought that whatever was happening was spread out all over my brain, but they didn't really explain why or how.

I started to think it might be something that runs in my family, like a genetic thing. My dad's side of the family had a cousin who also had seizures, but nobody really talked about it much. It's possible his seizures were caused by an injury, but it's hard to know for sure.

I recall a sense of frustration and confusion washing over me. It was like being handed a puzzle with crucial pieces missing. I yearned to understand why things unfolded the way they did, but sometimes the explanations remain elusive. It felt akin to staring at a blank page in a book—knowing that a story exists, yet unable to decipher it just yet.

Every few weeks, my grandma and I set off on a journey from our hometown of Lufkin, Texas, to the big city of Houston. It wasn't the most exciting trip, but we both knew it was necessary. I needed to see those doctors there who were experts at helping kids like me with epilepsy.

The drive felt really long, and sometimes it got a bit tiring. But I understood that we were doing it for a really good reason. When we finally reached the Houston Medical Center, I'd see families from all over the world. It made me realize how fortunate I was. Our drive was just a few hours, while some families traveled for days, even weeks, just to get there.

As I saw all those families from different places, my admiration for my grandma grew even stronger. Not once did she grumble about the long trips. She understood how crucial it was for me to receive the best care possible. And witnessing people come from all over the world to be there made me feel like I was in the perfect place, getting the finest help I could. Sure, it wasn't always easy, but it was absolutely worth it.

My grandparents watched over me as I grew up, showering me with love and support. They treated me just like any other kid, never making me feel fragile or different because of my condition. They urged me to explore, play, and learn without holding me back.

This approach truly molded my perspective on the world. I came to understand that when you try to protect someone excessively, even with the best intentions, it can inadvertently convey a message of incapability. The unwavering belief my grandparents had in me fostered a sense of confidence and independence that I continue to hold dear. It instilled in me the belief that, with the right support and mindset, there's no limit to what I can accomplish.

Although I considered myself a bit of a loner, my teenage years were still filled with fun times playing with my neighborhood friends. However, the years leading up to high school were a different story. I was never a very social person and only had one friend named Cy. He was a great athlete, and we always hung out together, but overall, life felt mundane.

After high school, Cy and I sought out opportunities to make some extra cash. We took on tasks like painting houses and mowing lawns. Then, we came across an unused house owned by Cy's grandpa in Lufkin. We made the decision to move in and start our own independent journey.

We used to have a blast fishing at Cy's grandpa's other house about 15 miles out of Lufkin. Around that time, I owned a pretty cool boat. Many of our friends also had boats and would often go water skiing.

Having been seizure free for awhile, I could still confidently drive a car and safely operate a boat. Achieving this gave me a strong sense of pride, knowing that I could carry out these tasks despite the challenges I had encountered earlier in life.

Chapter 4

Back then, my grandfather, Papaw, was my biggest fan. Every time I set foot on the baseball field, he was there in the stands, cheering me on. Sometimes, I must admit, I felt a little embarrassed. You see, he was older than most of the other kids' parents. I didn't quite realize at the time how extraordinary it was to have him there, supporting me with all his strength.

Only now, in retrospect, do I truly grasp the depth of that special bond we shared during those games. Now, I recognize the immense value of his presence. He made the effort to be there to back me up, regardless of his age. That's truly extraordinary. If I could turn back time, I'd tell my younger self to treasure those moments and understand just how much he cared about me and my games. It's a memory I'll forever hold dear.

Papaw, my mom's dad, deeply cherished cars. He devoted his days to managing his used car lot, where he would purchase and sell automobiles.

Occasionally, we'd embark on a journey to Tyler, Texas, for an auction, whether it occurred weekly or every other week. He was on the lookout for new cars, and I had the privilege of witnessing firsthand the entire process of acquiring and negotiating. Though it meant a bit of a drive, those trips transformed into days filled with shared adventures.

Once in a while, my grandma would join us too because she usually had a busy schedule during the week. In one particular instance, she came over, and Papaw was fully engrossed in negotiations, attempting to buy a used car. On the sidelines, Grandma and I decided to have some fun and began crafting a poem about astronauts. Eventually, NASA adopted our poem, making it their official piece for a flight in the late 1960s or early 1970s. It was a lighthearted endeavor, but it kept us happily occupied.

My family owned a plot of land just outside Tyler where we put a trailer home, a place we often called our weekend home. I personally undertook the task of cultivating a garden using a push plow, and it ended up becoming quite beautiful. I found the process not only rewarding but also a valuable learning experience.

In that same area, we were surrounded by extended family. They were heavily involved in haymaking, baling it up for storage. I occasionally joined in, stacking some bales in a nearby barn. It was fascinating to witness the entire process, from tending to the cattle to stacking the hay. I took joy in always being ready to lend a helping hand to my family members.

Reflecting on my past, I now understand that I've always cherished elderly individuals. Perhaps it's because they played such a significant role in my upbringing. Their wisdom and tales endlessly fascinated me. This early connection with them likely influenced my early aspiration to pursue a career in the medical field. I yearned to contribute, much like the remarkable individuals who molded my formative years.

When I turned 17, things took a scary turn. One normal day after school, I headed to my grandpa's used car lot. I knew he cherished his work there. Yet, upon arrival, my heart raced at the sight that met me.

Grandpa lay on the ground, appearing terribly ill; he had suffered a massive stroke. Two grown men stood nearby, looking bewildered. Without a moment's hesitation, I called the ambulance, stressing the urgency of our situation. They rushed over, swiftly administering oxygen to aid Grandpa's breathing.

The two men, one likely a coworker and the other a friend, seemed utterly lost and scared. I believe if I hadn't been there, we might have lost Papaw. It was an immensely trying moment, but I'm grateful I could step in.

As if things weren't already challenging enough, my world took a sharp turn when my grandfather had a stroke when I was just 17. Suddenly, everything seemed even more daunting. With my grandmother having no one else to turn to, a sense of responsibility washed over me. It became clear that I needed to step up and lend a hand in caring for him. It wasn't easy, but knowing how much my support meant to both of them made every effort worthwhile. This experience taught me the true meaning of family and the strength that comes from standing together in times of adversity.

I had finally got my driver's license when I was seventeen, and this was a major milestone for me. I was thrilled to be able to visit my paternal grandparents, who lived nine miles outside of Lufkin, Texas. People called the road McQueen's Hill, and it is still called that today. This newfound freedom behind the wheel was about to open up a whole world of possibilities, starting with this special visit to my grandparents.

Grandma McQueen, or Maggie, as I called her, was one of the most special people in my life. Despite being small in stature, all the other children in the family affectionately called her 'Big Mama'. Her love for gardening and canning pickles was something that always amazed me. She had the greenest thumb and was always eager to share her knowledge with anyone who would listen.

However, what stood out greatly about her was her incredible cooking skills. I looked forward to every mealtime because I knew that it was going to be something special. No one could cook quite like her. Her dishes were always filled with love, and even though I was young, I appreciated the time and effort she took to ensure that we were well fed and satisfied.

Every day, my cousins and I would gather at the table at precisely 5 o'clock, or we would risk missing out on her delicious cooking. It was a tradition we looked forward to and treasured.

Grandpa McQueen was one of the most influential people in my life. He taught me the value of hard work, which has been a constant driving force in my life. I remember spending countless afternoons with him on his land, helping him kill ants. He always paid me a nickel per ant bed, which might not have been much, but it taught me the importance of earning money through hard work.

On one occasion, he gave me a cow. He explained that he wanted me to have some money so I could sell the cow. So, we went to an auction with my cow my cow sold for a generous $1200 at the auction we went to, my grandpa handed the earnings to me. It was an enlightening process to be a part of, and I found it truly captivating.

Grandpa McQueen was also a pilot. We would spend time talking about flying and airplanes, and I was fascinated by his stories of adventure and exploration. One day, he took me up in his airplane, and we flew to Columbus, Texas. I remember feeling like I was on top of the world as we soared through the clouds and the thrill of being in control of such a magnificent machine.

As we flew, my grandfather let me take over the flying of the airplane. It was an incredible experience, and I felt like a true pilot, navigating the skies with ease. Though he was right there with me, guiding me every step of the way, I felt a sense of accomplishment and pride in my ability to fly an airplane at such a young age.

My grandfather had about a hundred acres of land. My daily routine involved going out there to chop wood, which was an activity that we both enjoyed. It was a great way to keep in shape, and I appreciate that he took the time to teach me a skill that I would carry with me for the rest of my life. Every evening, I would share supper with my grandparents, and once again, the food left me with a sense of home and warmth.

The lessons I learned from my grandfather have stayed with me to this day. His dedication to hard work and his passion for adventure have inspired me to chase my own dreams and embrace every opportunity that comes my way. And although he may no longer be with us, the memories of those afternoons spending time with him, fishing in his catfish ponds and soaring through the skies will always hold a special place in my heart.

My paternal grandparents had four daughters, and I was fortunate enough to have a wonderful relationship with each one of them. They were my aunts and were all unique, but they shared a common quality: they were kind, loving, and always made me feel welcome. Being surrounded by family who loved and cared for each other made this time in my life incredibly special. They taught me so much about love and what it meant to truly be there for those you cared about the most. I am forever grateful for the time I spent with my grandparents and my aunts.

Chapter 5

After graduating from high school, I reflected on my academic standing and realized that I had room for improvement. It made me feel quite disappointed in myself, but it motivated me to work harder and stay more dedicated to my studies. Looking back, I guess it was because I just didn't study enough and wasn't fully focused on my studies.

Nevertheless, I knew that I wanted to continue my education and pursue a career in pharmacy. So, I went directly to Angelina Junior College, just outside of Lufkin, to start my pre-pharmacy classes. I was in my 2nd year when they dropped my organic chemistry class because they didn't have enough registered students, as only 4 people had signed up for the class.

I then finished the year there and got my Associates Degree in Science (A.S.) and then went to a computer school in Dallas, TX, where I lived with my great-aunt Mitti for about 6 months. I got my Computer

Programmer Certificate, and that got me a job with some very talented computer programmers in Houston, Texas. I learned a lot from them. This job allowed me to further hone my new programming skills and develop a deeper understanding of computer technology. However, I still couldn't let go of my original dream of attending pharmacy school.

With my newfound confidence and a whole new set of skills under my belt, I decided to give pharmacy school another try. I applied in January 1985 to a professional pharmacy school. I was taken in after an interview and great reference letters, and I was thrilled to be accepted into the program. It was a competitive and challenging program, and I struggled initially. But I knew that I couldn't let my past academic struggles define my future.

I pushed myself harder than ever before, and I'm proud to say that I ultimately succeeded in pharmacy school. After almost failing in the first semester, I was able to turn things around and graduate with an impressive academic record. I realized that my experiences had taught me some incredibly valuable lessons about perseverance, grit, and determination, and I was grateful for the chance to prove to myself that I could succeed even when the odds were against me. It was a big shift, and it kept me pretty busy.

By now, my grandfather had been in bed for about 10 years, unable to talk or move much. He had to feed himself with his hands. My grandmother, too, went through a really tough time. She got something called Alzheimer's, which made it hard for her to remember things. It was hard to see my grandfather like that. He couldn't engage in the activities he once enjoyed, and communication became a struggle for him. On the other hand, my grandmother's memory continued to slip away, to the point where she sometimes didn't recognize me. It was truly heartbreaking to observe them both endure such hardships.

Within a span of merely three days, my dear grandfather and grandmother bid farewell to this world. It was the year 1986, and we held a joint funeral, a testament to the depth of their love. It was as if he couldn't bear to be apart from her. Their love story warmed my heart, and their absence was deeply felt. I hold onto the belief that they've embarked on a happier, pain-free existence together, in a realm far better than ours.

After their departure, life underwent a significant shift. Adjusting to their absence became a process that required time and understanding. At that point, I wasn't engaged in work, allowing me to be present with my family and properly mourn their passing. The emotions were a mix of sorrow and a peculiar sense of relief, knowing that they were no longer enduring pain. Honestly, their passing brought a feeling of relief. Witnessing their prolonged struggle, there was comfort in acknowledging that they had finally found peace. Regrettably, they weren't here to witness my graduation from pharmacy school.

Now, when I think of them, I remember the memories of the wonderful times we shared. My grandfather, Papaw, imparted invaluable life lessons, while my grandmother, Mamaw, filled my heart with her boundless love and selflessness. Their influence has played a significant role in shaping the person I've become. Though they've left this world, their love and our shared experiences remain etched in my heart. I believe they're looking down on me, and it's my deepest desire to live a life that would make them beam with pride.

I went back to school and worked hard. I resided approximately 35 miles from the University of Houston, my academic hub. Each morning, I embarked on the drive to campus. Classes commenced promptly at 8 a.m., making for a lengthy commute. Yet I recognized its value.

I was aware of the challenges that lay ahead. The rigorous curriculum, competitive admissions process, and demanding workload will require me to remain focused, disciplined, and dedicated. But I was confident in my ability to overcome these challenges and achieve my goals.

Back in pharmacy school, I had this really great friend named Peter. He came all the way from New Jersey. We spent a lot of time together, not just goofing off but also hitting the books. We would hang out and study together most of the time.

I graduated pharmacy school in May 1988 at the age of 29. After we both got our diplomas, Peter visited me at my place. He brought along his girlfriend, whom he eventually married. We all had a nice time hanging out. And even today, we're still in touch. It's pretty cool how strong friendships can last through the years.

When I graduated pharmacy school in 1988 at the age of 29, the world was a much different place than it is today. The United States was in the midst of Ronald Reagan's second term as president, and the country was experiencing a period of economic growth and prosperity. The Cold War was still ongoing, and tensions between the US and the Soviet Union were high.

The world of pharmacy was also vastly different in 1988. Pharmacies were predominantly run by independent, local pharmacists, and the use of technology in the field was still in its infancy. The concept of an "online pharmacy" had yet to be conceived, and the internet was still years away from becoming a mainstream tool for commerce.

After my graduation, my journey in the world of pharmacy began at a small store called Walgreens. I started as an intern. The boss, who was also a pharmacist, looked after the whole store, and I focused on running the pharmacy.

Back then, our store was the only one with a pharmacy. The doctor who wrote most of the prescriptions had really messy handwriting. He showed me how to figure out what he was writing, because if I could understand his handwriting, I could understand anyone's! The boss and I became really close friends during that time. We worked together closely and shared a great bond.

In the late 1980s, the pharmaceutical industry was undergoing significant changes. Various regulations were being put in place to ensure the safety and efficacy of prescription medications, making it more important than ever for pharmacists to have a deep understanding of the drugs they were dispensing.

Against this backdrop, I found myself preparing to take the registered pharmacist licensure exam in July 1988. Administered by the State of Texas, this comprehensive test was designed to evaluate my pharmaceutical knowledge across a wide range of topics. From drug interactions and side effects to dosage calculations and manufacturing processes, I was expected to have a thorough understanding of everything related to the practice of pharmacy.

Of course, passing the exam wasn't just a matter of memorizing facts and figures. I had to have a deep understanding of the underlying concepts and principles that informed the field. I needed to be able to think critically and apply my knowledge to real-world situations, whether I was helping a patient choose the right medication or collaborating with doctors to design treatment plans.

Against all odds, I passed the exam with flying colors. It was a defining moment in my career, marking the culmination of years of hard work and dedication to the field of pharmacy. With my new status as a registered pharmacist, I was ready to take on whatever challenges lay ahead, secure in the knowledge that I had the skills and knowledge needed to succeed in this fast-paced and constantly evolving industry.

I later went on to work at a different Walgreen store, which was pretty close to the one I worked at before. The boss there was a nice guy named Terry. When Halloween came around, he'd hand out candies and pencils to everyone. We got along well, and I even invited him over for dinner at my place once.

I was really into playing tennis, and Todd one of the workers at the front end of the store was studing to be an architect, which means he would designs buildings. After our shifts, we'd head to the tennis court and play. Let me tell you, he was amazing at it. He beat me every time, but it was a lot of fun trying to keep up with him.

There was one particular incident that stands out in my memory: the time when I had a seizure while at work. It all happened one day when a friend of mine and I were taking inventory at a pharmacy that I was working at. We had decided to go with a technician to help speed up the process. However, as the day wore on, I started feeling increasingly tired. Eventually, I succumbed to exhaustion and had a seizure without warning.

The result was catastrophic. I lost control of my body and fell into some of the shelving, causing an injury to myself that was not insignificant. My friend was immediately taken aback by what had happened, describing the situation as "scary." I can empathize with his fear, but for me, as an epileptic, experiences like this are not entirely unfamiliar.

Despite the challenges that come with being an epileptic or anyone with a chronic medical condition, you just keep going. You learn to persevere and not let setbacks define you. You acknowledge the hurdles, but you don't let them stop you from living your life to the fullest. While I have had to deal with more than my fair share of injuries and medical emergencies, I see each one as a challenge to overcome and a chance to grow stronger.

Chapter 6

In the midst of my life's journey, a wonderful person named Carol entered my world. She was a guiding light, brimming with love and friendship. Our paths converged, and through her, I discovered more than just a partner; she saw the strength within me.

Carol and I met on an online dating platform—a modern twist of fate that brought us together. Shortly after, we discovered that we lived just six miles apart, making the computer-mediated dating world seem unnecessary. We didn't talk on the computer anymore; we started talking on the phone, where we found ourselves lost in each other's words.

Over time, our relationship grew stronger. We shared our hopes, dreams, and fears with each other, and we picked each other up when we stumbled. Carol became my confidant, my supporter, and my partner.

From the beginning of our dating, I had disclosed my situation and told her I didn't want to burden her with it. However, she did not want to end the relationship on the basis of my epilepsy, and that made me love her even more.

One day, I mustered up the courage to ask Carol out for a meal. The prospect of asking her out made me a little nervous. I decided to playfully mention that I didn't own a car, only a tandem bicycle. Her response was unexpected and lighthearted, as she quipped, "That's perfectly fine, as long as you don't mind a female driver!" It was meant as a joke to gauge her reaction, as I did indeed have a car all along. The exchange added a touch of humor to the invitation, making it a memorable moment in our budding relationship.

Our first date was fantastic. Carol was not only delightful company but also incredibly sharp and captivating. Her intelligence and charm held my attention throughout the evening. We had decided on Babin's for our dinner, enjoying some delicious fish at that charming local restaurant. It was a wonderful start to what would become many more cherished moments together.

Our love story is a powerful example of how people connect. The things we went through together and the dreams we shared became the strong base of a partnership built on respecting and supporting each other. Together, we figured out how to go forward, facing life with a determined spirit to make a life full of happiness and meaning.

I was 43 years old when Carol and I got married. Before we tied the knot, I wanted to be honest with her. I reminded her about my epilepsy and said, "If you want me to, I'll walk away." But Carol looked at me and said, "You can't just get rid of me that easily."

So, on a warm June 15, 2002, we exchanged our vows and began this beautiful chapter of our lives together. Now, as I reflect on the years that have passed, I'm filled with gratitude that I didn't let fear or uncertainty hold me back from the love and partnership we share.

Carol's steadfast presence has been a source of strength and a reminder that love transcends any obstacle or challenge that life may throw our way.

When we started building our home together, it was clear that we clicked in more ways than one. From picking out paint colors to choosing furniture, we found ourselves on the same page about almost everything, agreeing about 95% of the time. It felt like our thoughts just naturally flowed together, like we were speaking the same language. This made the process not only enjoyable but also a true reflection of how well we understood each other. Building our home became a special journey that not only brought us closer but also showed us how in sync we really were.

We chose to hold off on our honeymoon, wanting to give it the extra special touch it deserved. After five years of patiently saving up, the moment finally arrived, and off we went to the beautiful shores of Barbados. It was an adventure filled with laughter, new experiences, and a deepening of our bond.

Fast forward another five years, and we found ourselves celebrating our 10th anniversary on the enchanting island of Bora Bora, just in time for Carol's birthday on June 29th. To mark this incredibly precious occasion, I had something truly magical in mind. A private dinner on the beach, with the sound of waves as our backdrop and the soft glow of candlelight, created an atmosphere that was nothing short of enchanting. Yes, it was a bit of a splurge, but the memories we made that evening were beyond measure. The look of joy and awe on Carol's face is something I'll carry in my heart forever. It was a moment that made every penny spent unquestionably worth it.

When Carol entered my life, she brought along a wonderful daughter, Christie. She was just 10 years old when we first met. Instantly, we connected over our shared passion for astronomy and mythology, something that Carol didn't particularly share.

Christie struggled with migraines, and many a night, I found myself awake at 2 a.m., doing my best to ease her pain. I was by her side, offering comfort and support. It was in those moments of vulnerability that our connection deepened.

Four years after we got married, I officially adopted Christie, and now she proudly carries my last name. I made sure to let her know that this decision was entirely hers to make, and when she did, I made it official.

This special addition expanded and strengthened our family in ways I couldn't have foreseen. I chose to Christie as an act of love that not only strengthened our ties but also reinforced the message that family is not solely defined by blood but by the bonds forged through love and shared experiences.

Carol is an amazing mom, and I always tried to do right by both of them, acting as the man of the house.

Their expressions of gratitude never failed to move me deeply. Knowing that I was making a positive impact simply by being myself brought me a profound sense of fulfillment and purpose.

Chapter 7

I had immersed myself in my studies, eager to learn all I could about the pharmaceutical industry. With each new lesson, I felt my passion and drive for this field grow stronger. My desire to help others achieve optimal health and wellness fueled my dedication to academics and motivated me to seek out opportunities to gain hands-on experience in various pharmacy settings.

Through internships and shadowing experiences, I witnessed firsthand the positive impact pharmacists can have on their patients' lives. These experiences solidified my decision to pursue a career in pharmacy and have further reinforced my commitment to making a positive difference in the lives of those around me.

I've learned that, in contrast to doctors, my job frequently calls for a more personal touch. Connecting with others on a level where they feel comfortable and understood has become a top goal for me. Beyond only issuing medications, my goal is to learn more about their worries and give them the assistance they require to feel in control of their healthcare journey.

I think that developing sincere connections with patients is essential to providing excellent medical services. It's basically providing a secure environment where they may freely express their concerns and queries. I try to decipher medical lingo through compassionate talks and provide simple, understandable explanations. People may confidently make educated decisions about their health in this way.

According to my observations, this strategy improves not only the patient-pharmacist interaction but also the overall results. Seeing the beneficial effects that a caring and understanding healthcare professional may have on a person's wellbeing is incredibly fulfilling. It confirms for me that medical science and compassionate care go hand in hand.

As someone who has always possessed a deep sense of compassion and a desire to alleviate the suffering of others, I have long been drawn to the field of healthcare. However, it wasn't until I began exploring the role of pharmacists in modern medicine that I realized this was the path I was meant to take.

What sets pharmacists apart from other healthcare providers is our hands-on approach to patient care. Instead of simply dispensing prescriptions and sending patients on their way, we take the time to establish personal connections with them. We listen to their concerns and offer advice on how to manage their conditions, providing not just medication but also guidance and support.

This personalized approach is what makes pharmacists more approachable than doctors and more reliable than pastors. Patients trust us to help them manage their conditions and improve their health, and we take this responsibility very seriously.

Becoming a pharmacist is more than just a career choice. It is a calling, a vocation, and a lifelong commitment to serving others. And I am grateful for the opportunity to pursue this path, to use my skills and knowledge to make a positive impact, and to honor the mentors who saw potential in me and encouraged me to follow my dreams.

I was fortunate to come across mentors on my journey who recognized the passion in my eyes and supported me in achieving my goals. One of them stands out—a pharmacist who is still a dear friend now. When I most needed help, this pharmacist, who is ten years older, lent a helping hand. He worked hard and put a lot of time into writing a letter of recommendation for me.

This seemingly insignificant act of compassion had a tremendous impact on my path. It served as the key to a future I had devoted my entire life to achieving. His encouragement not only confirmed my aspirations but also gave me new energy and direction.

I had a great desire to widen my professional horizons as the years passed. As a result, I went on to obtain more licenses in three other states: Oklahoma, Nevada, and Pennsylvania. I am now able to practice pharmacy in all four of these states because of the licenses I have acquired. This widened scope of work not only improved my career but also provided access to new encounters and contacts.

I've also added a significant duty as an immunizer since 2005. This implies that I get the privilege of giving immunizations, which are essential for preserving people's health and wellbeing. Being given this job is an enormous honor, and it makes me feel incredibly good to know that I'm personally improving people's lives.

Immunizing people involves more than just giving vaccinations; it also involves protecting communities, avoiding disease, and advocating for a healthier society as a whole. Each injection has the potential to protect people from a variety of diseases that can be prevented, perhaps saving lives and averting unnecessary suffering. Knowing that I am contributing to the creation of a world that is healthier and more resilient is a responsibility that I take seriously and carry out with determination.

My professional journey reached a crucial milestone in the year 2019. I earned certification in sterile compounding, a specialist area of pharmaceutical practice. This achievement signified a higher level of expertise and precision in the pharmaceutical industry.

The thorough production of drugs with a major focus on safety and accuracy is the core competency of sterile compounding. It includes a variety of procedures and methods to guarantee that each drug is not only efficient but also free from any impurities or toxins. In order to succeed in this specialized area of pharmacy, one must pay close attention to every last detail, adhere to all rules and regulations, and have a thorough understanding of the science involved in drug formulation.

Attending the American College of Apothecaries introduced me to the enriching world of extemporaneous compounding classes. This experience broadened my horizons and deepened my understanding of pharmaceutical compounding. Through rigorous coursework and hands-on training, I honed my skills in creating custom medicines to meet individual patient needs. These classes not only equipped me with technical expertise but also instilled in me a sense of precision and care in compounding medications. It was a transformative educational journey that has since played a pivotal role in shaping my career as a pharmacist.

While I haven't obtained certification in functional medicine just yet, I've been diligently studying it for a year and a half. It's a captivating field that focuses on using natural approaches to facilitate healing. Given my belief in the power of natural medicine, this is a pursuit I'm deeply passionate about.

What's truly remarkable is that I acquired some of my pharmacist licenses after turning 62 years old. This serves as a testament to the notion that one is never too old to continue learning and evolving. It's like catching a second wind in a race, and I'm still going strong!

When I graduated at 29 and became a pharmacist, I knew that I had made the right decision. Working in the healthcare sector was always a passion of mine, and I was excited to finally be able to use my skills and knowledge to help people in need. Little did I know, my journey was just beginning.

With each passing day, my determination burned brighter. Fueled by my experiences, I set my sights on a future as a pharmacist. The pursuit of this dream was no easy feat, but my unyielding resolve carried me through long hours of study, daunting exams, and countless moments of self-discovery. And in that journey, I emerged victorious, not just as a pharmacist but as a testament to the human spirit's capacity to overcome obstacles.

Balancing work and personal life can be quite a juggling act, especially for a pharmacist. The hours in this profession tend to be dynamic, ranging from the standard 9-5 to more unconventional shifts like 2-9. This variability can be a challenge, but it's also an integral part of the job. As a pharmacist, adapting to these changing hours becomes second nature. It's a testament to our flexibility and dedication to providing quality care to patients, no matter the time of day. So, while the schedule may be unpredictable, it's all part of the fulfilling journey of being a pharmacist.

Chapter 8

As days turned into years, my family continued to grow. The sound of our grandchildren's laughter and their pure innocence brought a new level of wonder to my journey. Through them, I've passed down crucial lessons about resilience and the importance of never giving up. I want them to hold onto the belief that they can conquer any obstacle and aim for the highest aspirations in life. They're like little stars, each with their own unique brilliance, capable of shining brightly.

During Christmas time, we go to our daughter's house to celebrate. We all come together at our place for Easter. My wife loves having everyone over, and our house is special because when you walk in, you can see all the way from the front to the back. We're lucky to have a pond behind our house, which adds to the fun. Kids especially enjoy it because they can go fishing. We even have a paddle boat and a kayak they can use. The grown-ups join in too, helping the kids with their fishing lines. It's a really wonderful time in my life. When everyone leaves, they're always happy, and their bellies are full of good food.

Our back porch is a special place for my wife. She enjoys spending time outdoors, and sometimes she even likes to sleep on the porch. To make it comfortable for her, I added a heater to the porch. It's a cozy spot where we can relax and enjoy the view of our ponds. It's her favorite place to be, and I wanted to make it perfect for her because I know how much she loves being outside.

Over the last 35 years, I have come across countless families that have been impacted by epilepsy. It has been heartbreaking to see the struggles that these families endure on a daily basis as they try to navigate a world where epilepsy is still not fully understood or accepted. However, what has been even more disheartening is when families feel powerless and helpless because of their child's diagnosis.

As I reflect on my life's path with epilepsy, I can't help but see how it's shaped me into who I am today. It's been a teacher of empathy, showing me the strength within compassion, and it's given me a resilience that I didn't know I had. It's a reminder that we all face our own battles, and it's those very struggles that build our strength.

Having challenges or disabilities is just a small part of the journey to achieving something great. I've faced tough times, but I've also learned that love, grit, and the support of family can be like a guiding light. They can help you find your way to a life that's not only successful but also deeply fulfilling.

Life is full of unexpected challenges that can test one's endurance and resilience. At times, it can feel like all hope is lost and that the hurdles presented in one's path are insurmountable. However, it is crucial to keep in mind that giving up is never the answer. Instead, it is imperative to face these obstacles head-on and persevere in the face of adversity. One must summon all their strength and unwavering determination to keep pushing forward.

It is essential to remember that real growth occurs in the midst of adversity. Overcoming challenges and rising above them is what makes us stronger and more resilient. It may be tempting to take the easy way out or to avoid the situation altogether, but this will only stunt one's growth and prolong the process of overcoming the challenge.

As a pharmacist, I have always believed that education is key when it comes to managing any condition or illness. This is especially true for epilepsy, where knowledge and understanding can make all the difference in the world. I have been fortunate enough to work with families who have been open and receptive to learning about epilepsy and who have been willing to put in the effort to help their child get their condition under control.

One thing that I always stress to these families is that having epilepsy does not mean that they are limited in any way. Yes, it is important to get the condition under control through medication and other treatments, but it should never hold anyone back from pursuing their dreams or aspirations. I have seen countless individuals with epilepsy go on to lead successful, fulfilling lives, whether it is in the arts, sports, or even as a pharmacist like myself.

At the end of the day, my message to anyone impacted by epilepsy is simple: don't let your diagnosis define who you are or what you can achieve. With the right mindset, education, and support, anyone can do anything they set their mind to.

Life is similar to climbing a mountain. Just like when scaling a mountain, there will be challenging moments where you might feel like giving up, but this is precisely when you must summon all your inner strength and push forward step by step. Although the top of the mountain may seem unreachable, it is attainable with each step taken and perseverance shown. When we finally reach the summit of our challenges, we find that it was all worth the struggle. In stepping up to face our problems, we emerge stronger and more capable of facing the next challenge that life may throw our way. Therefore, it is important not to let any hurdle hold us back and to continue to push through until we reach the top.

So, for anyone out there grappling with their own unique challenges, know this: You're not on this journey alone. Have faith in yourself, trust that every experience has a purpose, and let it guide you towards a place of inner fortitude, kindness, and self-discovery.

If you ever find yourself facing a challenge, remember that you're stronger than you think, and you've got a whole lot of love and support around you. That's the stuff that can turn a tough situation into a triumph. And that, my friend, is the secret to a truly meaningful life. This is what I've learned, and it's a lesson I carry with me every day.

About The Book

In "My Journey With Epilepsy Through Life," Michael McQueen shares with readers the details of his remarkable life, which is characterized by steadfast love, a strong will, and determination. Michael has struggled with epilepsy since he was ten years old, but with the unwavering love and support of his grandparents, he discovered that no hardship could ever define him.

From the peaceful surroundings of his childhood home to the fast-paced pharmacy industry, Michael's narrative exemplifies perseverance and a steadfast faith in the human spirit. He demonstrates that obstacles are only stop signs on the way to greatness with every victory against obstacles.

"My Journey With Epilepsy Through Life" is an inspirational narrative that goes beyond the limitations of ailment through heartfelt experiences and brilliant storytelling. For parents and kids struggling with epilepsy or any other difficulties, Michael's story offers hope and a reminder that they can accomplish anything they set their minds to.

This touching narrative is a testament to the power of love, family, and an unyielding spirit. Join Michael McQueen on a transformative journey that will leave you inspired to overcome any challenge life may present.

* 9 7 9 8 8 6 6 6 4 1 2 6 0 *